Chronic Pain

Chronic Pain

David J Rowbotham, MD, MRCP(UK), FRCA

Professor of Anaesthesia and Pain Management

University Department of Anaesthesia and Pain Management

Leicester Royal Infirmary

Leicester, UK

MARTIN DUNITZ

The views expressed in this publication are
those of the author and do not necessarily
reflect those of Martin Dunitz Ltd

First published in the United Kingdom in 2000 by
Martin Dunitz Ltd
The Livery House
7–9 Pratt Street
London NW1 0AE

Tel: +44 (0)207 482 2202
Fax: +44 (0)207 267 0159
E-mail: info@mdunitz.globalnet.co.uk
Website: http://www.dunitz.co.uk

A CIP catalogue record for this book is
available from the British Library

ISBN 1–85317–878–0.

Distributed in the USA, Canada and Brazil by:

Blackwell Science Inc.
Commerce Place, 350 Main Street
Malden MA 02148, USA
Tel: 1 800 215 1000

Printed and bound in Italy by Printer Trento S.r.l.

Contents

Pathophysiology of pain

Definitions

Many terms are used when describing the physiological and clinical aspects of pain, and there is often confusion as to their exact meaning. The most important of these terms, as defined by the International Association for the Study of Pain (IASP), are summarized in Table 1.

Pain is defined as 'an unpleasant sensory and emotional experience associated with actual or potential tissue damage, or described in terms of such damage'. Pain is a subjective sensation that is usually associated with tissue damage. However, some

Table 1 *Definitions of some pain terms*

Pain	An unpleasant sensory and emotional experience associated with actual or potential tissue damage, or described in terms of such damage
Allodynia	Pain due to a stimulus that does not normally provoke pain
Hyperalgesia	An increased response to a stimulus that is normally painful
Dysaesthesia	An unpleasant abnormal sensation, whether spontaneous or evoked
Paraesthesia	An abnormal sensation, whether spontaneous or evoked
Hyperaesthesia	Increased sensitivity to stimulation
Neuralgia	Pain in the distribution of a nerve

patients complain of pain in the absence of obvious damage or disease. In this situation, the symptom should still be regarded as pain even though the likely cause is psychological. The definition of pain is not dependent on an identifiable stimulus.

Chronic pain can be defined as pain persisting after the removal of, or in the absence of, a noxious stimulus. However, in some chronic pain syndromes the stimulus is constantly or intermittently present (e.g. pressure on a nerve by an intervertebral disk or cancerous tissue, or sickle cell crisis).

Peripheral nociceptors

A nociceptor is a receptor that is sensitive to noxious stimuli. Nociceptors are located at the terminals of afferent Aδ and C nerve fibres (Table 2). A noxious stimulus is one that is damaging to normal tissues. Aδ fibres are myelinated and transmit neural impulses relatively rapidly (at a rate of 10–40 m/second); C fibres are unmyelinated and transmit impulses slowly (at less than 2 m/second). High- and low-threshold nociceptors are attached to Aδ fibres, and they respond to mechanical and thermal stimuli. Those at the terminals of C fibres are high-threshold nociceptors, and they respond to thermal, mechanical and chemical stimuli.

Low-threshold touch receptors are located at the peripheral terminals of Aβ fibres. These fibres are myelinated and conduct impulses faster than Aδ and C fibres (i.e. at more than 40 m/second).

Table 2 *Primary nerve afferents responsible for pain*

Nociceptor	Speed/Sensation	Threshold	Stimuli
Aδ	10–40 m/second Sharp pain	High and low	Mechanical Thermal
C	<2 m/second Burning/itch	High	Mechanical Thermal Chemical

Nociceptors in the viscera are mostly attached to C fibres. These receptors respond to ischaemia, distension, excessive contraction of smooth muscle and chemical stimuli. Pain originating from the nociceptors tends to be perceived as dull, heavy or cramp-like.

Pain pathways

First-order afferent neurones have their nuclei in the dorsal root ganglia and synapse in the dorsal horn of the spinal cord (Figure 1). In general, nociceptor nerve fibres terminate in lamina I, II and V, from where the ascending pathways originate. (Lamina II is known also as the substantia gelatinosa.)

The most important ascending pathway is the spinothalamic tract, which is located anterolaterally in the spinal cord. After synapsing in the dorsal horn, most of the nerve fibres cross in the central white commissure of the spinal cord to enter the contralateral spinothalamic tract, eventually synapsing in the medial and lateral thalamus. Fibres from the lateral thalamus

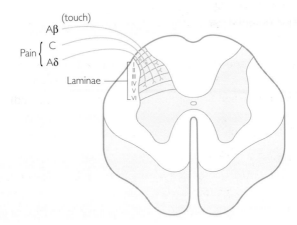

Figure 1 *Terminations of primary sensory afferents in the dorsal horn at the spinal cord.*

project into the sensory cortex and are probably responsible for the discriminatory and localizing character of pain. Some fibres that arise in the medial thalamus project to the periaqueduct grey matter, the reticular formation and the hypothalamus; these fibres are probably involved in the autonomic and emotional aspects of pain.

Two further ascending tracts are involved in transmission of pain. The spinoreticular tract terminates in the brain stem and medulla and the spinomesencephalic tract terminates in the mesencephalic reticular formation and the periaqueduct grey matter. Both of these tracts have ipsilateral and contralateral components.

In addition to ascending excitatory pathways, there are descending pathways in the dorsal columns of the spinal cord, which, when stimulated, inhibit the transmission of nociceptive signals in the dorsal horn.

Gate control theory of pain

The gate control theory of pain, introduced by Melzak and Wall, had a fundamental influence on the direction of basic research into pain and also on clinical management. The theory postulated that pain pathways in the spinal cord are modulated by inputs from other pathways (Figure 2). For example, rubbing a painful area stimulates Aβ fibres, which then inhibit the spinal synapses of Aδ and C fibres. Consequently, less input is delivered to the ascending pathways and less pain is perceived. The theory also speculated that higher centres could inhibit this system via descending pathways.

Perhaps the most important legacy of the gate theory is that it stimulated research into the identification of receptor systems and neurotransmitters involved in the mechanism of signal modulation. The expectation is that new drugs that act at these systems may soon be available for the treatment of pain. The theory

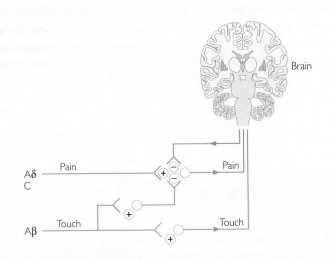

Brain

Aδ
C

Pain

Aβ

Touch

Pain

Touch

Figure 2 *Melzack and Wall gate control theory of pain. Pain pathways in the spinal cord can be inhibited by Aβ fibres via inhibitory spinal neurones or by inhibitory descending pathways (i.e. the pain gate is closed).*

also explains the action of transcutaneous electrical nerve stimulation (TENS) (see page 12) and spinal cord stimulation (see page 13) and gives a physiological basis for the efficacy of psychological techniques in reducing pain.

Hyperalgesia

Hyperalgesia (see Table 1) can be either primary or secondary.

Primary hyperalgesia

Primary hyperalgesia is defined as increased sensitivity to painful stimuli in an area of tissue damage or inflammation. An important mechanism for primary hyperalgesia is a reduction in nociceptor thresholds mediated by several locally acting substances, including prostaglandins. Non-steroidal anti-inflammatory drugs (NSAIDs) inhibit the production of prostaglandins (see page 19).

Other mediators include histamine, seretonin, hydrogen ions, bradykinin, calcitonin G-related peptide and cytokines.

Secondary hyperalgesia

Secondary hyperalgesia describes the phenomenon of increased sensitivity to painful stimuli in the normal healthy tissue that surrounds a damaged area (Figure 3). The area of secondary hyperalgesia increases rapidly with time after the initial injury but then declines as the noxious stimulus is removed. This response is known to be mediated in the spinal cord because it can be prevented by peripheral nerve blockade performed before application of the noxious stimulus.

It is postulated that, in many cases of chronic pain, the modified spinal cord function that is responsible for this normal response to acute injury does not return to normal. Therefore, patients continue to experience pain in and around tissue that is no longer receiving noxious stimuli. Mechanisms of secondary

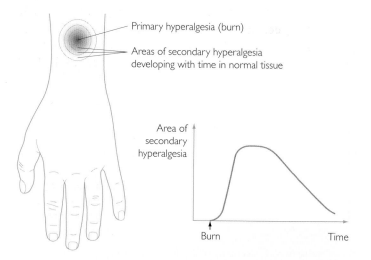

Figure 3 *Secondary hyperalgesia developing in a large area of normal tissue following a small burn.*

hyperalgesia include the involvement of intersegmental neurones and wide dynamic range neurones, the N-methyl D-aspartate (NMDA) and other receptors systems and changes in the phenotype of dorsal horn neurones. Wide dynamic range neurones receive input from C fibres that originate from a relatively large peripheral area. They may continue to discharge when C fibre input ceases.

Neuropathic pain

Broadly, there are two types of chronic or persistent pain (Figure 4). Nociceptive pain originates in the presence of normal pain pathways and tends to respond to standard analgesics. Neuropathic pain occurs when there is a functional or anatomical abnormality in the peripheral or central nervous system. It tends to respond poorly to standard analgesics.

Neuropathic pain may be described by the patient as burning, shooting or scalding. It is often accompanied by a history of nervous system insult and abnormal physical signs such as allodynia, sensory deficit and autonomic dysfunction. Common syndromes of neuropathic pain are described in Chapter 6. The pathophysiological causes are summarized in Table 3.

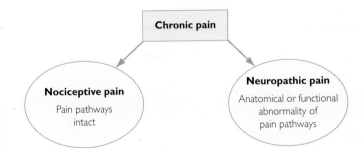

Figure 4 *The two types of chronic pain — nociceptive pain and neuropathic pain.*

Table 3 *Pathophysiological causes of neuropathic pain*

Spinal cord sensitization

Loss of inhibitory mechanisms

Ectopic neural activity

Sodium and calcium ion channel abnormalities

Migration of Aβ fibres into lamina I and II of the dorsal horn

Sprouting of sympathetic nerves around dorsal root ganglions

Catecholamine sensitivity

Neuropathic pain can also be described as sympathetically mediated if it responds to sympatholytic therapy or as sympathetically independent if it does not.

Further reading

Baranauskas G, Nistri A. Sensitization of pain pathways in the spinal cord: cellular mechanisms. *Prog Neurobiol* 1998;**54**:349–365.

Dickenson AH, Chapman V, Green GM. The pharmacology of excitatory and inhibitory amino acid-mediated events in the transmission and modulation of pain in the spinal cord. *Gen Pharmacol* 1997;**28**:633–638.

IASP Task Force on Taxonomy. *Classification of chronic pain*, 2nd edn. Seattle: IASP Press, 1994.

Raj PP. Pain mechanisms. In: Raj PP. *Pain medicine*. St Louis: Mosby, 1996 pp 12–25.

Willis WD, Westlund KN. Neuroanatomy of the pain system and of the pathways that modulate pain. *J Clin Neurophysiol* 1997;**14**:2–31.

Woolf CJ, Mannion RJ. Neuropathic pain; aetiology, mechanisms and management. *Lancet* 1999;**353**:1959–64.

Management options

The problem of chronic pain

Chronic pain is a major public health problem. It has significant and often devastating effects on well-being, quality of life and utilization of health care resources. In a recently published survey of a random sample of more than 5000 patients taken from the lists of general practitioners in the Grampian region of Scotland, the equivalent of 50.4% of the population reported chronic pain. Pain was described as 'high disability, severely limiting' in 15.8% of these patients who make enormous demands on the health-care system.

Many patients whose chronic pain responds to simple analgesics and who receive support from friends and family have a relatively good quality of life. However, a significant proportion do not respond to these measures and a specialist multimodal multidisciplinary approach is required if quality of life is to be maintained (Table 4). In this chapter, the types of management available for chronic pain are summarized. The pharmacological treatment of pain is expanded on in this book but, for more detail on other modalities, the reader is referred to the further reading list at the end of this chapter.

Drug treatment

For most patients, the mainstay of treatment is pharmacological (see Chapters 3, 4 and 5). In general:

Table 4 *Treatment modalities for chronic pain*

Drugs
Analgesics
Antidepressants
Anticonvulsants
Miscellaneous
Nerve blocks
Temporary
Permanent
TENS
Implantable devices
Pumps
Dorsal column stimulation
Psychological therapies
Education
Relaxation
Diversion
Operant behavioural techniques
Cognitive behavioural techniques
Stress management
Physiotherapy
Exercises
Electrical stimulation (e.g. inferential therapy)
Ultrasound
Pulsed shortwave
Heat
Massage
Manipulation
Complementary therapies
Acupuncture
Hypnotherapy
Reflexology
Homoeopathy
Aromatherapy
Shiatsu

TENS, transcutaneous electrical nerve stimulation.

- nociceptive pain responds to paracetamol, NSAIDs and opioids; and
- neuropathic pain to antidepressants, anticonvulsants and other drugs.

It cannot be emphasized too much that drugs may only reduce pain and may fail to relieve it completely. Other measures may be required to translate reduction in pain severity to improved quality of life.

Oral medication is the preferred route of administration for most patients, and many analgesics are available in a sustained-release formulation that provides a steady background blood concentration. However, other modes of administration can be used to improve analgesia. For example, in severe pain, opioids may be delivered directly into the cerebrospinal fluid or the epidural space. Fentanyl (an opioid agonist; see page 35) is available in a patch formulation for transdermal administration. Other modes of administration include intravenous, lingual, rectal and intramuscular. Any of these may be appropriate in specific situations.

Nerve blocks

Single-shot blocks
Nerve blockade with a local anaesthetic is used extensively in the management of chronic pain. A nerve block can help in the diagnosis (e.g. pain in the lateral aspect of the thigh that is relieved completely by a block of the lateral cutaneous nerve of the thigh is highly suggestive of neuralgia of that nerve). Local anaesthetic blocks, often mixed with a corticosteroid preparation (e.g. methylprednisolone), are often used with therapeutic benefit.

Infusion techniques
Prolonged blockade can be achieved by continuous infusion of local anaesthetic via a catheter inserted adjacent to the nerve.

For example, a catheter can be placed in the brachial sheath in order to produce prolonged analgesia of the arm. Postoperative analgesia by epidural is a commonly used example of this technique.

Permanent blocks

The axonal sheath of a nerve can be disrupted leading to long-lasting blockade if substances such as ethanol or phenol are injected. This technique is commonly used to produce a permanent chemical lumbar sympathectomy (e.g. in sympathetically maintained leg pain) or a coeliac plexus blockade (e.g. in carcinoma of pancreas). The most important complication of this technique is motor nerve damage. Nerves can also be destroyed with radiofrequency lesions (e.g. facet nerve ablation for back pain), cryolysis or surgery.

Transcutaneous electrical nerve stimulation

Transcutaneous electrical nerve stimulation (TENS) inhibits the 'pain gate' in the spinal cord by stimulating Aβ nerve fibres (see page 5). A small battery-powered device delivers electrical current (usually 0–80 mA) to one pair of pad electrodes applied to the skin or to two pairs of electrodes (dual output). Traditional TENS ('Hi TENS') utilizes a frequency of approximately 100 Hz and a narrow pulse width. A lower frequency (2–5 Hz) is used in 'Lo TENS'. In addition to the background stimulation, TENS can be applied as a brief, intense stimulation during periods of severe pain.

TENS is widely used in chronic pain therapy. It is simple and has few side effects. However, the patient needs to understand that pain relief will often be experienced only during treatment. TENS can be very effective but it is best used as part of a comprehensive management plan that involves other modalities of treatment as well. In some patients, TENS is completely ineffective and may increase pain.

Implantable devices

Implantable devices can be helpful in severe cases of chronic pain. Infusion pumps are able to deliver drugs (e.g. opioids) spinally to provide excellent analgesia while allowing the patient to be mobile and at home. Dorsal column stimulation involves the insertion of a small signal generator attached to an electrode, which is placed in the epidural space. The electrode inhibits the pain gate by stimulating the descending inhibitory tracts in the dorsal columns of the spinal cord. This technique requires considerable expertise and rigorous patient selection.

Psychological management of pain

The basis behind the psychological management of pain is the inhibition of the 'pain gate' by higher centres in the brain via the inhibitory descending pathways in the spinal cord. Factors that may open and close the gate are shown in Figure 5.

It should be remembered that a psychological approach to chronic pain is absolutely vital if maximum success is to be achieved. The brief description here does not reflect its importance and efficacy. Many psychological techniques are available, and patients with significant chronic pain should ideally be assessed by a clinical psychologist. However, simple techniques

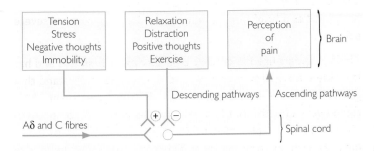

Figure 5 *Psychological factors affecting the 'pain gate'.*

such as counselling and education can be performed by all suitably trained health-care professionals.

Education
The knowledge and understanding that patients have about their condition often affects their perception of pain and their response to it. For example, a patient who believes that back pain represents a worsening of pathology will not mobilize well and the pain will have a significant effect on quality of life. Education helps patients to adapt to their condition.

Relaxation
Relaxation techniques decrease central arousal and muscle tension and often improve symptoms. They may give the patient a greater sense of self-control.

Diversion techniques
Diversion techniques decrease perception of pain by teaching patients to switch their attention to other stimuli.

Operant behavioural techniques
Operant behavioural therapy involves setting specific goals in a step-like fashion. Patients' positive behaviour towards achieving these goals are reinforced by staff.

Cognitive behavioural techniques
The basis of the cognitive behavioural approach is that the emotional and behavioural response to pain is influenced primarily by thoughts (e.g. beliefs and expectations) rather than by the disease process itself. The aim is to change these thoughts and, consequently, the response to pain.

Stress management
Stress management techniques may be appropriate in some patients.

Pain management programmes

Psychological techniques may be applied during individual or group sessions. However, for some patients, a pain management programme is appropriate. Pain management programmes are usually led by psychologists but outcome is improved if a multi-disciplinary approach is used. Programmes often last for 3–4 weeks and patients may be resident or attend daily. All relevant psychological approaches are used in combination with supervised exercises and goal setting.

Physiotherapy

The physiotherapist has expertise in the assessment of musculo-skeletal conditions and will often help with diagnosis as well as management. The physiotherapist can be a vital member of the multidisciplinary team. The goal of chronic pain management is to improve quality of life, which is linked intimately with mobility and function. Any improvement in pain that results from treatments such as injections or drugs can be translated into improved function by physiotherapy.

Several physiotherapy techniques can provide analgesia, including:

- electrical stimulation (e.g. inferential therapy);
- ultrasound;
- pulsed shortwaves;
- heat;
- massage; and
- manipulation.

Complementary therapies

Acupuncture

Although not considered as mainstream conventional therapy, acupuncture it is widely available. Many patients appear to receive significant benefit from acupuncture, but its precise efficacy in chronic pain states is yet to be determined. The principles behind acupuncture are not those of Western medicine, and the location of needle points does not relate to the anatomy of the peripheral nervous system. Traditional Chinese acupuncture involves over 300 needle points situated along meridians. As well as the use of classical fine acupuncture needles that are manipulated by hand, acupuncture can be applied using electrical stimulation, by blunt pressure (e.g. sea bands for travel sickness) and, more recently, by laser stimulation.

Other complementary therapies
Several other therapies are available (e.g. chiropractic, hypnotherapy, reflexology, homoeopathy, aromatherapy and shiatsu), but there are no clear indications of their efficacy. Despite this, some patients derive great benefit from them.

Further reading

Ashburn MA, Staats PS. Management of chronic pain. *Lancet* 1999;**353**:1865–1869.

Becker N, Bondegaard TA, Olsen AK, Sjogren P, Bech P, Eriksen J. Pain epidemiology and health related quality of life in chronic non-malignant pain patients referred to a Danish multidisciplinary pain center. *Pain* 1997;**73**:393–400.

Burton HJ, Kline S, Hargadon R, Shick R, Ong M, Cooper B. Chronic pain patients' quality of life improves with increased life control. *Pain Clin* 1998;**11**:33–42.

Crosbie J, McConnell J, eds. *Key issues in musculoskeletal physiotherapy.* Oxford: Butterworth Heinmann, 1994.

Elliott AM, Smith BH, Penny KI, Smith WC, Chambers WA. The epidemiology of chronic pain in the community. *Lancet* 1999;**354**:1248–1252.

Ernst E. Massage therapy for low back pain: a systematic review. *J Pain Symptom Management* 1999;**17**:65–69.

Feine JC, Lund JP. An assessment of the efficacy of physical therapy and physical modalities for the control of musculoskeletal pain. *Pain* 1997;**5**:5–23.

Fischer HJ. Peripheral nerve blockade in the treatment of pain. *Pain Rev* 1998;**5**:183–202.

Fishbain DA, Cutler R, Rosomoff HL, Rosomoff RS. Chronic pain-associated depression: antecedent or consequence of chronic pain? A review. *Clin J Pain* 1997;**13**:116–137.

Gureje O, Von Korff M, Simon GE, Gater R. Persistent pain and well-being: a World Health Organization study in primary care. *JAMA* 1998;**280**:147–151.

Guthrie E. Emotional disorder in chronic illness: psychotherapeutic interventions. *Br J Psychiatry* 1996;**168**:265–273.

Hill PA, Hardy PJ. The cost-effectiveness of a multidisciplinary pain management programme in a district general hospital. *Pain Clin* 1996;**9**:181–188.

Hojsted J, Alban A, Hagild K, Eriksen J. Utilization of health care system by chronic pain patients who applied for disability pensions. *Pain* 1999;**82**:275–282.

Jonson MI, Ashton CH, Thompson JW. An indepth study of long-term users of transcutaneous electrical nerve stimulation: implications for the clinical use of TENS. *Pain* 1991;**44**:221–229.

Lamacraft G, Molloy AR, Cousins MJ. Peripheral nerve blockade and chronic pain management. *Pain Rev* 1997;**4**:122–147.

Loeser JD. Economic implications of pain management. *Acta Anaesthesiol Scand* 1999;**43**:957–959.

Malone MD, Strube MJ. Meta-analysis of non-medical treatments for chronic pain. *Pain* 1988;**34**:231–244.

Morley S, Eccleston C, Williams A. Systematic review and meta-analysis of randomized controlled trials of cognitive behaviour therapy and behaviour therapy for chronic pain in adults, excluding headache. *Pain* 1999;**80**:1–13.

Nurmikko TJ, Nash TP, Wiles JR. Recent advances: control of chronic pain. *BMJ* 1998;**317**:1438–1441.

Portenoy RK. Opioid therapy for chronic non-malignant pain: a review of the critical issues. *J Pain Symptom Management* 1996;**11**:203–217.

Savage SR. Opioid use in the management of chronic pain. *Med Clin North Am* 1999;**83**:761–786.

Turk DC, Okifuji A. Efficacy of multidisciplinary pain centres: an antidote to anecdotes. *Baillières Clin Anaesthesiol* 1998;**12**:103–119.

Vaarwerk IM, Staal MJ. Spinal cord stimulation in chronic pain syndromes. *Spinal Cord* 1998;**36**:671–682.

Waldman SD, Winnie AP, eds. *Interventional pain management.* Philadelphia: WB Saunders, 1996.

Ward D. *TENS clinical applications and related theory.* Edinburgh: Churchill Livingstone, 1997.

Non-steroidal anti-inflammatory drugs and paracetamol

Non-steroidal anti-inflammatory drugs

Mechanism of action

Non-steroidal anti-inflammatory drugs (NSAIDs) decrease the production of prostaglandins by inhibiting the enzyme cyclo-oxygenase (COX) (Figure 6). It can be seen that COX acts early in the chain of events (i.e. well before prostaglandin receptor activation), and thromboxane and prostacyclin synthesis is inhibited by NSAIDs as well as prostaglandins. This relatively non-specific action is responsible for the analgesic, antiplatelet, antipyretic and anti-inflammatory effects of NSAIDs (Table 5).

Two types of COX have been identified (COX 1 and COX 2). COX 1 is a 'house-keeping' enzyme (i.e. it is present in most tissues and is involved with routine activities). In particular, it is

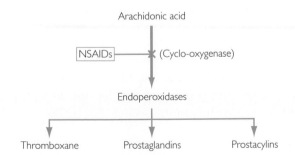

Figure 6 *Action of NSAIDs in inhibiting the enzyme cyclo-oxygenase, thereby leading to a decrease in prostaglandin synthesis.*

Table 5 *Activity of NSAIDs acting at COX 1 and COX 2 (non-specific COX inhibitors)*

Analgesia

Anti-inflammatory effects

Anti-pyretic effects

Gastric ulceration and bleeding

Anti-platelet effects

Impairment of renal function (especially if dehydrated)

Exacerbation of asthma in some patients

COX, cyclo-oxygenase; NSAID, non-steroidal anti-inflammatory drug.

involved with prostaglandin synthesis in the gastric mucosa and renal vascular bed as well as with thromboxane A_2 synthesis in platelets. Inhibition of COX 1 is responsible for side effects such as gastrointestinal ulceration, bleeding and impaired renal function. COX 2 is produced at sites of inflammation and is not present in platelets or gastric mucosa. However, it is normally present in the central nervous system. Inhibition of COX 2 leads to analgesia and anti-inflammatory effects.

Pharmacodynamics
All NSAIDs that have been available for prescription until recently inhibit COX 1 and 2. Consequently, their pharmacodynamics are very similar. However, the incidence of side effects differs between drugs, perhaps as a result of differences in the specific activity of each drug against the COX 1 and COX 2 enzyme. The drugs can be classified with respect to their likelihood of producing gastric erosions (Table 6). Ibuprofen is less likely than other NSAIDs to produce gastric erosions, but the incidence of this problem with other frequently used NSAIDs is similar.

Pharmacokinetics
NSAIDs are absorbed well after oral administration, are highly albumin-bound and most have short half-lives (2–3 hours).

Table 6 *Relative risk of adverse gastric side-effects with NSAIDs (non-specific COX inhibitors)*

High risk
Azapropazone
Moderate risk
Diclofenac
Ketoprofen
Indomethacin
Naproxen
Piroxicam
Low
Ibuprofen

Data from Committee on the Safety of Medicines (CSM) and published reports.
COX, cyclo-oxygenase; NSAID, non-steroidal anti-inflammatory drug.

However, several are available in slow-release preparations and some have long half-lives, especially the oxicams. Drug interactions can be a problem with NSAIDs, often because they displace other drugs from albumin sites and increase the free plasma concentration of these other drugs. Some important interactions are shown in Table 7.

Individual NSAIDs

Despite having similar properties, there are probably more NSAID preparations available in the UK than there are for any other class of drug. However, the NSAID preparations are very similar and only a brief summary can be given here.

Aspirin (acetysalicylic acid) is metabolized to salicylic acid. At moderate to high doses, there is a high incidence of side effects and, because of the association with Reye's syndrome, it is contraindicated in children. Diflunisal is also metabolized to salicylic acid but it is more potent and has a longer duration of action than aspirin.

Table 7 *Drug interactions with NSAIDs*

Drug	Effect
ACE inhibitors Therapy for cardiac failure	Hypokalaemia
Potassium-sparing diuretics Anti-hypertensive agents	↓ Effectiveness, sodium and water retention
Lithium	↑ Plasma lithium
Methotrexate	↑ Free plasma methotrexate concentration
Phenytoin	↑ Free plasma phenytoin concentration
Tolbutamide	Hypoglycaemia
Warfarin	↑ Free plasma warfarin concentration

ACE, angiotensin converting enzyme; NSAID, non-steroidal anti-inflammatory agent.

Diclofenac is a phenylacetic acid derivative. It is available as oral, rectal and intramuscular preparations. The intramuscular preparation is associated with a high incidence of pain at the injection site.

Many NSAIDs are proprionic acid derivatives (e.g. ibuprofen, ketoprofen, fenoprofen, naproxen, fenbufen) and are used widely. They all have very similar pharmacological properties.

Indomethacin is a methylated indole derivative and has a relatively high incidence of side effects, particularly gastrointestinal side effects.

Sulindac is a derivative of indomethacin and is popular because it is believed to be safer in patients with impaired renal function.

Ketorolac was developed for the treatment of postoperative pain and can be given either intramuscularly or intravenously.

The oxicam group of NSAIDs tend to have prolonged half-lives; examples are piroxicam, which has a half-life of 50 hours, and tenoxicam which has a half-life of 72 hours.

Many NSAID creams are available and are often used for musculo-skeletal complaints. They are not devoid of gastric side effects.

Use of NSAIDs in acute pain

NSAIDs are often used in the management of acute pain, especially pain after surgery. Many patients with chronic pain require surgery, and NSAIDs are usually continued over the peri-operative period. During this time, the antiplatelet and renal effects become more important because of the potential increased risk of perioperative bleeding and the increased likelihood of de-hydration and sodium depletion leading to renal failure.

The Royal College of Anaesthetists have published guidelines on the use of NSAIDs in the perioperative period and some of the recommendations are shown in Table 8. It is recommended that

Table 8 *Recommendations of the Royal College of Anaesthetists on the peri-operative use of NSAIDs (non-specific COX inhibitors)*

Situations in which NSAIDS should be avoided	Situations in which NSAIDs should be used with caution
Past history of gastrointestinal bleeding or ulceration	Elderly patients
Renal impairment	Asthma
Hypovolaemia	Diabetes mellitus
Hyperkalaemia	Widespread vascular disease
Aspirin-sensitive asthma	Cardiac, hepatobiliary, vascular surgery
Severe liver dysfunction	Concomitant administration of:
Uncontrolled hypertension	ACE inhibitors
	Potassium-sparing diuretics
Pre-eclamptic toxaemia	Beta Blockers
Systemic inflammatory response syndrome	Cyclosporin
	Methotrexate
Circulatory failure	

ACE, angiotensin converting enzyme; NSAID, non-steroidal anti-inflammatory drug.

renal function should be monitored regularly after major surgery in all patients who are receiving NSAIDs and that the NSAIDs should be stopped if urine output decreases or if plasma electrolytes suggest the development of renal impairment.

COX 2-specific NSAIDs

Any drug that inhibits COX 2 but not COX 1 should be an analgesic and an anti-inflammatory agent with no effects on the gastric mucosa or platelets. This theory has led to the development and recent introduction for clinical use of the COX 2-specific NSAIDs.

Celecoxib and rofecoxib are the first available COX 2-specific NSAIDs and it is likely that more will follow. Early data suggest that, compared with non-specific COX inhibitors, COX 2-specific inhibitors are associated with similar analgesia and anti-inflammatory effects but have no effect on platelets or gastric mucosa (Table 9). However, effects on renal function and in patients with asthma are not yet clear.

COX 2-specific inhibitors are likely to play a major role in the management of many chronic pain conditions.

Table 9 *Comparison of specific COX 2 inhibitors with non-specific COX inhibitors (early impressions)*

Similar analgesia

Similar anti-inflammatory effect

No effect on platelets

No effect on gastric mucosa

Renal effects—uncertain

Effects on patients with asthma—uncertain

COX, cyclo-oxygenase.

Paracetamol

The mechanism of action of paracetamol (acetaminophen) remains one of the unsolved mysteries of modern medicine. However, it is known to reduce prostaglandin concentrations in the brain. Paracetamol has no significant effect on peripheral COX enzymes and no anti-inflammatory activity and it does not cause gastric ulceration. However, it is an effective analgesic and antipyretic agent.

Unfortunately, because of its widespread availability, the efficacy of paracetamol is often not appreciated either by patients or health-care workers. Used regularly, and in combination with NSAIDs or opioids, paracetamol can significantly improve pain relief in many chronic pain conditions. The major problem with paracetamol is that it may cause fatal hepatic necrosis if taken in overdose.

Further reading

Atcheson R, Rowbotham DJ. Pharmacology of acute and chronic pain. In: Rawal N, ed. *Clinical acute and chronic pain.* London: BMJ Publications, 1998.

Brouwers JJ, Desmet PM. Pharmacokinetic–pharmacodynamic drug interactions with non-steroidal anti-inflammatory drugs. *Clin Pharmacokin* 1994;**27**:462–485.

Emery P, Zeidler H, Kvien TK, *et al.* Celecoxib versus diclofenac in long-term management of rheumatoid arthritis: randomised double-blind comparison. *Lancet* 1999;**354**:2106–2111.

Fenner H. Differentiating among non-steroidal anti-inflammatory drugs by pharmacokinetic and pharmacodynamic profiles. *Semin Arthritis Rheum* 1997;**26**:28–33.

Moore RA, Tramer MR, Carroll D, Wiffen PJ, McQuay HJ. Quantitive systematic review of topically applied non-steroidal anti-inflammatory drugs. *BMJ* 1998;**316**:333–338.

Rodriguez LG. Non-steroidal anti-inflammatory drugs, ulcers and risk: a collaborative meta-analysis. *Semin Arthritis Rheum* 1997;**26**:16–20.

Royal College of Anaesthetists. *Guidelines on the use of non-steroidal anti-inflammatory drugs in the perioperative period*. London: Royal College of Anaesthetists, 1998.

Schafer AI. Effects of non-steroidal anti-inflammatory drugs on platelet-function and systemic hemostasis. *J Clin Pharmacol* 1995;**35**:209–219.

Scott LJ, Lamb HM. Rofecoxib. *Drugs* 1999;**58**:499–505.

Willett LR, Carson JL, Strom BL. Epidemiology of gastrointestinal damage associated with non-steroidal anti-inflammatory drugs. *Drug Safety* 1994;**10**:170–181.

Wolfe MM, Lichtenstein DR, Singh G. Gastrointestinal toxicity of non-steroidal anti-inflammatory drugs. *N Engl J Med* 1999;**340**:1888–1899.

Opioid analgesics

Familiarity with the definitions listed in Table 10 is important for the understanding of opioid pharmacology. Opium is obtained from the seeds of the poppy plant *Papaver somniferum* ('opion' means 'poppy' in Greek). Raw opium consists of over 25 opioids but morphine is the most important constituent (making up 9–17%). However, many opioids in clinical use are either entirely synthetic (e.g. pethidine and fentanyl) or are derived from naturally occurring opiates (e.g. diamorphine (diacetyl-morphine)).

Table 10 *Definitions in opioid pharmacology*

Opioid	Any drug acting at an opioid receptor
Opiate	A naturally occurring opioid (e.g. morphine, codeine)
Efficacy	Maximum effect of a drug
Potency	Dose required to produce 50% of maximum effect (i.e. ED_{50})
Agonist	A substance that binds to a receptor mediating an intracellular response
Pure agonist	An agonist that can produce the maximum response that the receptor is capable of mediating
Partial agonist	An agonist the maximum response of which is less than that of a pure agonist
Antagonist	A substance that binds to a receptor but does not mediate a response

Opioid receptors

Five types of opioid receptors were described in the 1970s (μ, κ, σ, δ and ϵ) but it rapidly became apparent that only three of these (μ, κ, and δ) were true opioid receptors. These three receptors are all involved in analgesia but the μ-receptor is thought to be primarily responsible for respiratory depression and constipation. Dysphoria is particularly associated with κ-receptor agonists.

Opioid receptors are found in the dorsal horns of the spinal cord (especially lamina I and the substantia gelatinosa). They inhibit the release of neurotransmitters from the presynaptic terminal (by inhibiting calcium channels) and inhibit depolarization of the postsynaptic membrane (by enhancing potassium channels).

Efficacy and potency

The terms 'efficacy' and 'potency' are often confused (see Table 10).

> The efficacy of a drug is the value of its maximum effect.

For example, with respect to effects on respiratory function, morphine has the same efficacy as pethidine (i.e. both can cause respiratory arrest). Buprenorphine does not normally cause respiratory arrest and therefore it is less efficacious than either morphine or fentanyl. The same comparison can be made for degree of analgesia.

> The potency of a drug is the dose required to produce 50% of the maximum response (i.e. the ED_{50}).

Therefore, morphine is more potent than pethidine. Compared with both morphine and pethidine, buprenorphine is more potent since a typical dose of buprenorphine may be 0.3–0.6 mg.

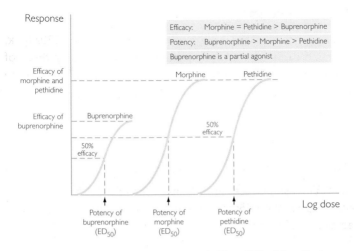

Figure 7 *Efficacy and potency of three opioids. ED_{50}, 50% of the effective dose.*

Figure 7 illustrates the relationship between potency and efficacy using the dose–response curves of morphine, pethidine and buprenorphine.

Classification of opioids

Traditionally, opioids have been classified as strong, intermediate or weak, according to their perceived analgesic properties (Table 11).

Table 11 *Traditional classification of opioids*

'Weak' opioid	'Intermediate'-strength opioids	'Strong' opioids
Codeine	**Partial agonists**	Morphine
	Buprenorphine	Diamorphine
	Mixed agonists–antagonists	Pethidine
	Pentazocine	Fentanyl
	Butorphanol	
	Nalbuphine	

Although this classification has been useful, it can be misleading. For example, codeine (a 'weak opioid') is simply less potent than morphine (i.e. a greater dose is required for the same effect). However, codeine can still lead to respiratory depression if it is given in a sufficient dose.

Intermediate opioids include partial μ-receptor agonists (which have less efficacy than morphine) and mixed agonist–antagonists (i.e. compounds that act as **antagonists** at the μ receptor but as **agonists** at the κ receptor). They are seen as intermediate because they are weaker analgesics than morphine but they are potentially useful because they are less likely to be associated with respiratory depression and addiction. However, nausea, sedation and dysphoria are often troublesome.

A more functional classification of opioids is shown in Table 12.

Table 12 *Functional classification of opioids*

Pure agonists (full agonist at the opioid receptors only)
Morphine, diamorphine, fentanyl
Partial agonist
Buprenorphine
Mixed agonist-antagonists (κ-receptor agonist and μ-receptor antagonist)
Pentazocine, butorphanol, nalbuphine
Mixed-action drugs (possess pharmacological activity other than opioid)
Pethidine (anticholinergic, local anaesthetic), tramadol (inhibits uptake of noradrenaline and 5-HT)
5-HT, 5-hydroxytryptamine (serotonin).

Effects of opioids

Most opioids have very similar pharmacodynamic effects (Table 13). Any differences usually result from pharmacokinetics or activity at non-opioid sites.

Apart from analgesia, the most important effects of opioids include:

- respiratory depression;
- sedation;
- nausea and vomiting; and
- constipation.

Tolerance to all of these effects occurs, and many patients with cancer pain may be receiving relatively enormous doses of opioids and yet remain alert. However, tolerance to constipation

Table 13 *Common effects of opioids*

Central nervous system effects
Analgesia
Sedation
Nausea and vomiting
Meiosis
Euphoria
Dysphoria
Respiratory effects
Respiratory depression
Cardiovascular effects (usually after overdose or rapid injection)
Hypotension
Bradycardia
Gastrointestinal side effects
Delayed gastric emptying
Constipation

is infrequent and this is often the dose-limiting factor in chronic opioid therapy.

Pharmacokinetics of opioids

Most opioids have poor oral bioavailability (Table 14). Methadone is an exception and is absorbed almost completely after oral administration. Despite this, and although bioavailability varies greatly between patients, the oral route is still preferred by most patients with chronic pain. When changing to and from other methods of administration (e.g. intramuscular, intravenous, subcutaneous or transdermal), it is important to take the oral bioavailability into account.

The plasma half-lives of some commonly used opioids are shown in Table 15. Most have relatively short half-lives, so regular doses or sustained-release preparations are required for prolonged effects. The duration of action of some opioids is longer than their half-life would suggest because of active metabolites (e.g. morphine and diamorphine) or high receptor affinity (e.g. buprenorphine). Methadone, however, has a long half-life; it can

Table 14 *Oral bioavailability of some opioids*

Opioid	Oral bioavailability (%)
Codeine	50
Hydromorphone	30
Methadone	92
Morphine	25
Nalbuphine	16
Oxycodone	60
Pentazocine	47
Pethidine	52
Tramadol	75

Table 15 *Plasma half-lives of some opioids*

Opioid	Plasma half-life (hours)
Alfentanil	1.6
Codeine	2.9
Fentanyl	3.5
Hydromorphone	3.1
Methadone	20–45
Morphine	3
Nalbuphine	2.3
Oxycodone	3.7
Pentazocine	4.6
Pethidine	4
Tramadol	7

be taken once per day but it takes many days before a steady-state plasma concentration is achieved.

Individual opioids

Morphine
Morphine (named after Morpheus, the Greek god of dreams) was first isolated from opium in 1806. Its major metabolites are morphine-6-glucuronide and morphine-3-glucuronide, which are excreted in urine and accumulate in renal insufficiency. Morphine-3-glucuronide is inactive but morphine-6-glucuronide is a potent agonist at the μ-receptor.

Diamorphine
Diamorphine (3,6-diacetyl morphine; heroin) is synthesized from morphine and has no activity at the μ-receptor. It is a prodrug and is converted rapidly to its active metabolite 6-monoacetyl morphine, which is metabolized further to morphine. There is a

common belief that that diamorphine is associated with more euphoria and less nausea and vomiting than morphine. It has been shown clearly that this is not so—diamorphine has no advantages over morphine.

Codeine

Codeine (3-methoxy morphine) is also a prodrug with no activity at the opioid receptor. About 10% of a dose is metabolized in the liver to morphine by the polymorphic enzyme CYP2D6, which is absent in some people (e.g. 7% of Caucasians). This may account for the ineffectiveness of this drug in some patients.

Pethidine

Pethidine (meperidine) has a shorter duration of action than morphine. Most of its metabolites are inactive but one of them (norpethidine) causes excitation of the central nervous system, which leads eventually to convulsions. Convulsions are more likely after prolonged and high-dose administration.

Pethidine is contraindicated in patients who are currently taking monoamine oxidase inhibitors (MAOIs) and in those who have received them within the past 2 weeks. This is because of irreversible enzyme inhibition. Reactions can be excitatory (delirium, rigidity, hyperpyrexia and coma) or inhibitory (respiratory and cardiovascular collapse and coma). Pethidine is a poor choice for chronic pain.

Hydromorphone

Hydromorphone is a semisynthetic opioid. It is approximately six times more potent than morphine. In contrast to morphine, there are no significantly active metabolites.

Oxycodone

Oxycodone is also a semisynthetic opioid. When given as a sustained-release oral preparation, it is approximately twice as potent as morphine.

Fentanyl

Fentanyl is approximately 100 times more potent than morphine, has no active metabolites and is comparatively short-acting. It can be given transdermally for the management of chronic cancer pain.

Methadone

Methadone is a synthetic opioid with a high oral bioavailability and a long duration of action (it has a half-life of 20–45 hours). It can be given once daily but steady-state plasma concentrations may not be reached for 10 days. Presently, its use in cancer and other chronic pain states is increasing because of the suggestion that methadone may inhibit spinal cord 'wind-up' by acting as an antagonist at the NMDA-receptor.

Tramadol

Tramadol is a relatively weak μ-receptor agonist but it is metabolized into o-desmethyltramadol, which has greater affinity for the receptor. It also inhibits noradrenaline and serotonin (5-hydroxytryptamine, 5-HT) uptake, which probably increases descending inhibitory tone on the spinal cord. Therefore, tramadol may cause analgesia by acting at two distinct sites.

Buprenorphine

Buprenorphine is a partial μ-receptor agonist with a high receptor affinity. It is not so effective as morphine, has a relatively long duration of action and can be given sublingualy. Although less likely to cause respiratory depression it causes constipation, nausea and vomiting.

Mixed agonist–antagonist opioids

Drugs in this class include pentazocine, butorphanol and nalbuphine. Despite being μ-receptor antagonists, they cause analgesia because they are κ-receptor agonists. Analgesic efficacy is poor compared with pure μ agonists but they have less effect on respiratory function. Unfortunately, dysphoria and nausea are relatively common side effects.

Tolerance, dependence and addiction

Appropriate use of opioids for chronic pain is often confounded by a profound misunderstanding of tolerance, dependence and addiction by patients and health-care workers.

> Tolerance occurs frequently with opioid therapy—it refers to the need to administer increasing doses of a drug in order to obtain the same effect.

> Dependence is a state in which an abstinence syndrome may occur following abrupt opioid withdrawal or administration of an opioid antagonist.

Dependence is often confused with addiction. Many patients who are dependent on opioids are able live a normal and useful life—they are not opioid addicts. Addiction (as defined by the World Health Organization) is characterized by compulsive self-administration of a drug on a continuous or periodic basis in order to experience its psychic effects and to avoid discomfort caused by its absence, with supply often being secured by deceptive or illegal means. Addiction is extremely rare in patients receiving opioids for chronic pain relief if they are managed by specialists. Indeed, it is more common in those prescribing the medication than those who are receiving it. Addiction is not an issue in patients with terminal cancer but it is a potential problem in non-cancer states. Opioids can be used successfully in patients with a long life-expectancy, but the drugs should be administered by specialists in accordance with well-accepted guidelines.

Further reading

Atcheson R, Rowbotham DJ. Pharmacology of acute and chronic pain. In: Rawal N, ed. *Clinical acute and chronic pain*. London: BMJ Publications, 1998.

Cherny NI. Opioid analgesics. Comparative features and prescribing guidelines. *Drugs* 1996;**51**:713–737.

Fine FG. Fentanyl in the treatment of cancer pain. *Semin Oncol* 1997;**24**:20–27.

GilmerHill HS, Boggan JE, Smith KA, Wagner FC. Intrathecal morphine delivered via subcutaneous pump for intractable cancer pain: a review of the literature. *Surg Neurol* 1999;**51**:12–15.

Kirkpatrick AF, Derasari M, Kovacs PL, Lamb BD, Miller R, Reading A. A protocol-contract for opioid use in patients with chronic pain not due to malignancy. *J Clin Anesth* 1998;**10**:435–443.

McQuay HJ. Opioid use in chronic pain. *Acta Anaesthesiol Scand* 1997;**41**:175–183.

Payne R. Factors influencing quality of life in cancer patients: the role of transdermal fentanyl in the management of pain. *Semin Oncol* 1998;**25**:47–53.

Portenoy RK. Opioid therapy for chronic nonmalignant pain: a review of the critical issues. *J Pain Symptom Management* 1996;**11**:203–217.

Ripamonti C, Zecca E, Bruera E. An update on the clinical use of methadone for cancer pain. *Pain* 1997;**70**:109–115.

Savage SR. Opioid use in the management of chronic pain. *Med Clin North Am* 1999;**83**:761–786.

Antidepressants, anticonvulsants and other drugs

Neuropathic pain does not respond well to standard analgesics (NSAIDs, paracetamol and opioids). However, symptoms may respond to other drugs that were not originally intended to be used as analgesics but have subsequently been found to be of use in neuropathic pain. The mainstays of such therapy are antidepressants (especially amitriptyline) and anticonvulsants. Some drugs have been given indications for use in neuropathic pain associated with specific diseases, but several others have not. Gabapentin is the only drug that is licensed in the UK for the treatment of neuropathic pain *per se*.

The following drugs and drug classes are used for their analgesic effects in certain circumstances:

Antidepressant agents
Anticonvulsant agents
Antiarrhythmic agents
Capsaicin
Baclofen

Antidepressant agents

Antidepressants have specific analgesic effects, for which they are often prescribed in small doses. They inhibit the uptake of noradrenaline and 5-HT in the spinal cord, enhancing the inhibitory effects of the descending spinal pathways. Amitriptyline is the antidepressant that is most often prescribed, but others such as desipramine, imipramine and doxepin are used by some practitioners. In contrast to amitriptylene, desipramine inhibits noradrenaline reuptake more than 5-HT reuptake, but the clinical relevance of this difference is uncertain.

Many patients with chronic pain become clinically depressed, and antidepressant medication is clearly indicated in this situation to improve mood. This indication should not be confused by healthcare workers or patients with the use of these drugs for pain relief. The theory behind the use of antidepressants for analgesia must be explained in simple terms to patients. If they are prescribed with no explanation, many patients will think that the doctor simply does not believe that they are in pain and that all their symptoms are caused by depression. Consequently, the patient will not take the medication and will be denied a chance of significant pain relief.

Amitriptyline

Amitriptyline is a tricyclic antidepressant that is readily absorbed after oral administration. It is metabolized in the liver to its main active metabolite, nortriptyline. It is extensively bound to plasma and tissue proteins (the volume of distribution is 10–50 litres/kg) and it has a long, variable half-life (9–25 hours). It has no license for pain relief but the literature confirms its effectiveness. In practice, side effects (particularly sedation but also dry mouth, constipation, agitation and confusion) often limit its use. However, if amitriptyline is given at night, the sedative effect can be very helpful to those patients with disturbed sleep.

For analgesia, many practitioners prescribe amitriptyline 10 mg at night, increasing to 20 mg after 1 week. This is well below the recommended starting dose for treatment of depression (50–100 mg in young adults). If side effects are not troublesome, it can be given twice daily or at higher doses. Some patients will report sedation or dry mouth that was associated with previous administration of high-dose amitriptyline. In this situation, the use of low-dose amitriptyline should be considered.

Anticonvulsant agents

Anticonvulsants affect the function of neuronal ion channels and stabilize neuronal membranes by a variety of mechanisms, some of which are still to be elucidated. Mechanistically, these drugs should be effective in some types of neurogenic pain, and clinical practice confirms this.

Gabapentin

Two large studies have shown the efficacy of gabapentin for the pain of postherpetic neuralgia and diabetic neuropathy, and there is a growing body of evidence in the literature suggesting efficacy in various types of neuropathic pain. Indeed, gabapentin has recently been given a licensed indication by the Committee for the Safety of Medicines in the UK for the treatment of neuropathic pain and should be titrated to a maximum dose of 1800 mg/day.

Gabapentin is virtually unbound (less than 3%) to plasma proteins. It is not metabolized and is excreted unchanged by the kidneys. The half-life is approximately 6 hours. It is reasonably well tolerated, but side effects include sedation, dizziness, ataxia, headache and nausea. There is no need to monitor blood counts or plasma concentrations of gabapentin routinely during therapy, and there are relatively few potential drug interactions.

Carbamazepine

Carbamazepine can be effective in neuropathic pain, especially trigeminal neuralgia, for which it is licensed. It is well absorbed orally (the bioavailability is 85–100%), is 75% protein-bound and has an active metabolite (carbamazepine epoxide). The half-life during regular administration is 16–24 hours.

The dose required to control neuropathic pain varies widely. Treatment should be commenced with a small dose (e.g. 100 mg twice daily in the elderly) and the dose gradually increased. Often pain is controlled with 200 mg three or four times daily but the dose can be increased gradually to 1600 mg daily.

However, efficacy is often limited by side effects such as gastro-intestinal upset, headaches, confusion, visual disturbances and rash. Agranulocytosis and aplastic anaemia have been reported, and it is recommended that blood counts should be taken before, and at intervals during, treatment with carbamazepine.

Phenytoin

Phenytoin is an anticonvulsant with a licence for the treatment of trigeminal neuralgia in patients in whom carbamazepine is ineffective or not tolerated. It is well absorbed after oral administration and is highly protein bound with a very variable half-life (7–42 hours). This variable half-life, plus the fact that phenytoin is metabolized by zero-order kinetics, leads to large changes in free plasma concentrations in response to both relatively small changes in dose and interactions with other drugs. It is recommended that treatment is monitored by regular measurement of plasma phenytoin.

Side effects include rashes of various types (including exfoliative dermatitis, Stevens–Johnson syndrome), hyperglycaemia, cerebellar dysfunction, abnormal facial features such as gum hyperplasia and hirsutism, sedation, confusion and various haematological problems. As a result of these side effects, phenytoin is prescribed infrequently for neuropathic pain.

Sodium valproate

Sodium valproate is well absorbed orally and metabolized extensively in the liver. It is occasionally used to treat neuropathic pain but has no licence for this indication. Side effects include gastrointestinal upset, rashes, ataxia, tremor, liver dysfunction and thrombocytopenia. Fatal liver failure has been reported and the manufacturers recommend that liver function tests should be performed before, and at intervals during, therapy, especially in children, who are most at risk of liver problems.

Lamotrigine

Lamotrigine is well absorbed after oral administration, weakly (55%) protein-bound in the plasma, extensively metabolized and has a long half-life (24–35 hours). Side effects include headache, sedation, rash, dizziness and insomnia. Efficacy in some types of neuropathic pain has been reported.

Antiarrhythmic agents

Intravenous infusion of lignocaine (at doses up to the maximum recommended dose) is occasionally used for the treatment of neuropathic pain. This should be performed under careful monitoring by practitioners who are experts in cardiovascular resuscitation.

Benefit from intravenous lignocaine is often short-lived. Therefore, if analgesia is produced by an intravenous infusion, oral mexiletine is occasionally prescribed in order to obtain a longer-term effect. However, its use is limited by the by the relatively frequent incidence of troublesome side effects such as nausea, gastrointestinal upset, dizziness and palpitations.

Capsaicin

Capsaicin is the active constituent of chilli peppers. It is available as a cream, which is licensed for pain associated with post-herpetic neuralgia and diabetic neuropathy. It has been postulated that capsaicin stimulates continuously peripheral nociceptors, thus depleting stores of neurotransmitters that enhance transmission in the pain pathways. A sensation of warmth or burning is experienced when the cream is applied to the affected area of skin, particular during the early stages of treatment. Repeated application is associated with desensitization and inhibition of C-fibre conduction, but maximum effects may not be observed for 6–8 weeks. Capsaicin can be very effective, but some patients refuse to use the cream because of the painful, burning sensation.

Baclofen

Baclofen is indicated for the relief of spasticity of voluntary muscles, which is often painful. It can be given orally but its use may be limited by side-effects, including sedation, confusion, dizziness, insomnia, decreased convulsion threshold, muscle weakness, ataxia and psychiatric disorders. Baclofen can be administered intrathecally by an implantable programmable pump, but this should be performed in specialist centres.

Further reading

Backonja M, Beydoun A, Edwards KR, et al. Gabapentin for the treatment of painful diabetic neuropathy in patients with diabetes mellitus. *JAMA* 1999;**280**:1831–1836.

Di Vadi PP, Hamann W. The use of lamotrigine in neuropathic pain. *Anaesthesia* 1998;**53**:808-809.

McQuay H, Carroll D, Jadad AR, Wiffen P, Moore A. Anticonvulsant drugs for management of pain: a systematic review. *BMJ* 1995;**311**:1047–1052.

McQuay HJ, Tramer M, Nye BA, Carroll D, Wiffen PJ, Moore RA. A systematic review of antidepressants in neuropathic pain. *Pain* 1996;**68**:217–227.

Rowbotham M, Harden H, Stacey B, Bernstein P, Magnus-Miller L. Gabapentin for the treatment of postherpetic neuralgia. A randomized controlled trial. *JAMA* 1999;**280**:1837–1842.

Spina E, Pisani F, Perucca E. Clinically significant pharmacokinetic drug interactions with carbamazepine: an update. *Clin Pharmacokin* 1996;**31**:198–214.

Common chronic pain syndromes

Principles of management

The first task in the management of patients with chronic pain is to make a diagnosis. The diagnosis may be obvious, as in post-herpetic neuralgia or postsurgical phantom limb pain, but occasionally it is difficult. Detailed history, examination, investigation and referral to appropriate specialists will facilitate diagnosis. However, a precise diagnosis may not be possible. If this is so, and before embarking upon symptomatic pain management, it must be ensured that all reasonable attempts have been made to make a diagnosis. Pain experienced by patients in whom diagnosis is difficult should be managed just as aggressively as that experienced by patients in whom a diagnosis has been made.

Occasionally, one treatment modality alone relieves the symptoms of a chronic pain condition. However, more often than not, several modalities are necessary and a multidisciplinary approach with an emphasis on improving quality of life is required (see Chapter 2). If possible, patients should be referred to a pain clinic, many of which offer this multidisciplinary approach.

Broadly, chronic pain syndromes can be divided into nociceptive and neuropathic conditions.

Nociceptive complaints include common conditions such as:
- back and neck pain;
- musculoskeletal pain;
- headaches;
- osteoarthritis;

- rheumatoid arthritis;
- post-surgical and trauma pains; and
- chronic pain that arise from the viscera and pelvis.

It is not possible to discuss the detailed management of all these conditions here. In general, the approach is to optimize analgesic therapy (e.g. choice of drug, mode of administration, titration of dose) and to use other treatment strategies (e.g. nerve blocks, TENS, acupuncture, physiotherapy, psychology), as described in Chapter 2.

Neuropathic pain

The characteristics of neuropathic pain have been described in Chapter 1. Neuropathic pain arises because of an abnormality in the nervous system and it can be extremely severe and have devastating effects on quality of life; it is sometimes difficult to treat.

Complex regional pain syndrome (CRPS)

Definitions

The term 'complex regional pain syndrome' (CRPS) represents a relatively new nomenclature introduced by the International Association for the Study of Pain (IASP) in an attempt to simplify a confusing picture. Terms often used to describe this condition are listed in Table 16. Reflex sympathetic dystrophy (RSD), causalgia, algodystrophy and Sudeck's atrophy are terms that are still in common use.

The IASP has defined two types of CRPS. CRPS type 1 (formerly RSD) develops after a noxious event and is not limited to the distribution of a single peripheral nerve. The IASP diagnostic criteria are shown in Table 17. CRPS type 1 is associated with oedema, changes in skin blood flow, abnormal sudomotor activity and allodynia or hyperalgesia. The IASP criteria for the diagnosis of CRPS type 2 (causalgia) are listed in Table 18. It is associated with burning pain and allodynia after partial injury of a nerve.

Table 16 *Terms commonly used to describe complex regional pain syndrome (CRPS)*

Reflex sympathetic pain syndrome

Causalgia

Algodystrophy

Sudeck's atrophy

Sympathetically maintained pain

Post-traumatic dystrophy

Shoulder–hand syndrome

Table 17 *IASP diagnostic criteria for complex regional pain syndrome type 1 (reflex sympathetic dystrophy). Criteria 2–4 must be satisfied*

1. Initial noxious event or cause of immobilization
2. Continuing pain, allodynia or hyperalgesia with pain disproportionate to the inciting event
3. Evidence at some time of oedema, changes in skin blood flow or abnormal sudomotor activity in the region of pain
4. The diagnosis is excluded by the existence of conditions that would otherwise account for the degree of pain or dysfunction

IASP, International Association for the Study of Pain.

Table 18 *IASP diagnostic criteria for complex regional pain syndrome type 2 (causalgia). All criteria must be satisfied*

1. The presence of continuing pain, allodynia or hyperalgesia after a nerve injury, not necessary limited to the distribution of the nerve
2. Evidence at some time of oedema, changes in skin blood flow or abnormal sudomotor activity in the region of pain
3. The diagnosis is excluded by the existence of conditions that would otherwise account for the degree of pain and dysfunction

IASP, International Association for the Study of Pain.

Sympathetically maintained pain may be associated with CRPS and is characterized by symptomatic relief after sympatholytic interventions (e.g. guanethidine block or sympathetic blocks).

Clinical symptoms and signs

Clinically, three phases of CRPS have been described. In the acute stage, patients complain of severe pain (often burning or shooting) associated with allodynia or hyperalgesia, or both. Symptoms may develop after minor injury. The skin may be warm and well perfused or, particularly towards the end of this phase, cyanosed and cold. Oedema and severe limitation of movement is common.

At this stage, symptoms and signs may resolve spontaneously or after treatment. However, it often progresses to the second (dystrophic) phase, which is characterized by increased pain, allodynia and hyperalgesia. The skin becomes cold and poorly perfused, often with decreased hair and nail growth. Oedema increases and movement and power of associated muscle groups decrease. At this stage, osteoporosis begins to be detectable by X-ray.

The final, atrophic phase may accompanied by a decrease in the intensity of pain, but many patients continue to experience agonizing neuropathic pain with intense allodynia. The disease process spreads further and may involve the whole limb. Tissues become atrophied and joints become fixed with flexor contractures. Not surprisingly, psychological disturbance often becomes prominent.

Management

Early detection and specialist referral is essential. Too many patients with CRPS are referred for specialist treatment at stages when changes have become irreversible. Good-quality studies in this difficult patient population are lacking and there is no accepted ideal management protocol. Treatment options include:
- optimal analgesia with opioid and non-opioid analgesics, tricyclic antidepressants and anticonvulsants;

- intravenous guanethidine blocks;
- sympathetic blockade; and
- physiotherapy (utilizing optimal analgesia).

In the later stages, psychological support and comprehensive rehabilitation is indicated. Neurostimulation and acupuncture have also been used.

Phantom limb pain

Phantom limb pain (a sensation of pain arising from an area or the whole of an amputated limb) should be distinguished from non-painful phantom sensation and nociceptive pain arising from the stump. Phantom limb sensation is a normal event but patients should be warned of the likelihood of this before surgery or immediately after trauma. Psychological support may be required to help the patient to come to terms with this situation. Stump pain is common immediately after surgery but its severity should decline rapidly. Causes of persistent stump pain include:
- poorly fitting prostheses;
- ischaemia;
- myofascial trigger points;
- osteomyelitis; and
- peripheral nerve neuromas.

The literature is inconsistent with respect to the incidence of phantom limb pain, but some authorities have quoted an incidence of about 85%. In general, the incidence and severity decreases with time, but a significant number of patients are left with severe incapacitating pain many years after amputation. In some patients the pain is constant; in others it is episodic—often stimulated by physical activity or emotional distress. Pain in an amputated limb may be particularly distressing for some patients and they need reassurance that they are not imagining their symptoms. Patients with troublesome persistent phantom limb pain benefit from comprehensive multidisciplinary pain management.

Symptomatic improvement has been reported with the use of:

- drugs (particularly antidepressants and anticonvulsants);
- TENS;
- physiotherapy techniques;
- nerve blocks;
- acupuncture; and
- psychological approaches.

Refashioning of the stump may be indicated if non-invasive techniques are unsuccessful and if the stump is in some way deficient (e.g. because of ischaemia or palpable neuromas).

Postherpetic neuralgia

Postherpetic neuralgia occurs after an episode of acute herpes zoster infection (shingles) resulting from a reactivation of the chickenpox virus, which remains dormant in the dorsal root ganglion. However, pain usually settles when the rash heals. Postherpetic neuralgia has been defined as pain that continues 1 month after the disappearance of the rash. The pain of postherpetic neuralgia can be very severe and distressing and can have a devastating effect on quality of life. Patients often complain of a constant burning pain with episodes of severe shooting pain occurring either spontaneously or on minimal stimulation of the affected skin.

Pharmacological therapy includes:

- tricyclic antidepressants;
- anticonvulsants;
- sympathetic block; and
- capsaicin or local anaesthetic cream.

Trigeminal neuralgia

Trigeminal neuralgia is another intensely painful example of neuropathic pain. Classically, the patient experiences periods of intense, sharp, stabbing pain interspersed with pain-free periods. Stimuli that may trigger pain include light touch, cold air and eating. Pain is restricted to the area innervated by the trigeminal nerve, especially the mandibular and maxillary divisions. Apart from trigger points, neurological examination is normal. Before the diagnosis is made, other causes of facial pain should be eliminated by careful examination and investigation.

Pain may be relieved by antidepressants or anticonvulsants, or both. Other treatments include trigeminal ganglion blocks (by alcohol or radiofrequency lesions) and psychological approaches. Neurosurgery (vascular decompression of the trigeminal nerve via a posterior fossa approach) can be curative in a significant number of patients. Any patient with symptoms suggestive of trigeminal neuralgia should be referred for specialist attention as soon as possible.

Painful peripheral neuropathies

Peripheral neuropathies are characterized by a loss of sensation (touch, pain, vibration and position) commencing in the feet or hands. They may be associated with dysaesthesias and, despite detectable loss of sensation, they may be painful. Causes of painful peripheral neuropathy include:

- diabetes mellitus;
- rheumatoid arthritis;
- myeloma;
- leukaemia;
- alcoholism;
- vitamin deficiency; and
- drugs.

It is essential to seek a diagnosis in this situation because pain often improves if the underlying cause is treated. Otherwise, pain management is broadly similar to that of other neuropathic pain syndromes.

Compression neuropathies

Neuropathic pain can be caused by compression of a nerve or nerve root. Common causes include a prolapsed intervertebral disc and degeneration or collapse of the spinal root canal. Surgery may be indicated, especially if there is motor nerve involvement, but non-surgical management is often appropriate. Pharmacological treatment is similar to that of other types of neuropathic pain, but a multidisciplinary approach to the problem is usually essential.

Post-traumatic neuropathic pain syndromes

Nerves may be damaged during trauma or surgery. Nociceptive pain associated with fractures and wounds subsides but neuropathic pain arising from damaged nerves often does not.

Further reading

Allen G, Galer BS, Schwartz L. Epidemiology of complex regional pain syndrome: a retrospective chart review of 134 patients. *Pain* 1999;**80**:539–544.

Bowsher D. Trigeminal neuralgia: an anatomically oriented review. *Clin Anat* 1997;**10**:409–415.

Cluff RS, Rowbotham MC. Pain caused by herpes zoster infection. *Neurol Clin* 1998;**16**:813–835.

Green MW, Selman JE. The medical management of trigeminal neuralgia (review article). *Headache* 1991;**31**:588–592.

Hill A. Phantom limb pain: a review of the literature on attributes and potential mechanisms. *J Pain Symptom Management* 1999;**17**:125–142.

IASP Task Force on Taxonomy. *Classification of chronic pain*, 2nd edn. Seattle: IASP Press, 1994.

Kingery WS. A critical review of controlled clinical trials for peripheral neuropathic pain and complex regional pain syndromes. *Pain* 1997;**73**:123–139.

Tekkok IH, Brown JA. The neurosurgical management of trigeminal neuralgia. *Neurosurg Q* 1996;**6**:89–107.

Cancer pain

Fortunately, most patients with cancer do not suffer from severe intractable pain. Pain in cancer is usually controlled by proper use of oral analgesics (NSAIDs, paracetamol and opioids). However, some patients require specialist pain management in order to control their symptoms. In patients with cancer, pain is only one aspect of management and, ideally, patients should have access to palliative care physicians, nurses and other specialists. The approach to pain management in the terminally ill can differ from those patients who have a normal life expectancy. The use of opioids can be more liberal and techniques of analgesia that are complicated and are associated with potentially serious side effects become more appropriate (e.g. chronic spinal opioid administration, ablative nerve blocks).

> Every modality of pain relief discussed in this book can be used in patients with cancer, and the importance of the holistic approach cannot be over-emphasized.

Specific syndromes in cancer pain

Severe pain in cancer is usually associated with cancerous tissue in bones or invasion of nervous tissue by tumour. Bony metastasis can cause severe pain or lead to painful pathological fractures. Vertebral metastases can cause structural collapse, which may compress spinal nerves or even the spinal cord, leading to neuropathic pain as well as motor abnormalities.

Direct involvement of the nervous system can give rise to several syndromes. Tumours may invade individual peripheral nerves or the cervical, brachial or lumbar plexuses, and pain may be aggravated by venous obstruction and lymphoedema. Invasion of the coeliac plexus is common in pancreatic tumours and this is responsible for one of the most distressing pain syndromes. Involvement of the spinal cord meninges is associated with numerous unpleasant signs and symptoms, many of which are painful.

Antitumour treatments can sometimes be responsible for troublesome pain. For example, many patients with cancer undergo major radical surgery and may suffer from chronic postsurgical pain. Radiotherapy can cause neuralgia (e.g. brachial neuralgia after radiotherapy for breast cancer), and chemotherapy can induce painful neuropathies.

Management

Oral analgesia

Opioids are the mainstay of therapy but it should be remembered that regular NSAIDs and paracetamol also have a useful role to play. It is important to titrate opioid dose to effect, and large doses may be required because of tolerance. If tolerance becomes a problem, many clinicians change to another opioid in an attempt to improve efficacy. As yet, there is little scientific evidence for this. Methadone has become popular because of its possible action at the NMDA receptor. Whatever the opioid, therapy should be tailored precisely to symptoms, and this is often achieved by using a combination of sustained-release and rapidly absorbed preparations.

Pethidine is best avoided because accumulation of its metabolite (norpethidine) may cause tremors or convulsions. Background analgesia with fentanyl can be provided reliably by the transdermal method.

Spinal opioids

Intraspinal administration of opioids can be very effective in patients in whom oral therapy is unsatisfactory. Local delivery of opioid can be delivered directly to the opioid receptors in the spinal cord producing profound analgesia with little sedation. A catheter is placed at the appropriate vertebral level in the cerebrospinal fluid or epidural space and the drug is delivered by an external or implanted pump. If managed with care, this technique can be very effective.

Antidepressants and anticonvulsants

If neuropathic pain is a problem, standard analgesics are not likely to be helpful. Antidepressants or anticonvulsants, or both, should be prescribed.

Nerve blocks

Nerve blocks with local anaesthetics and corticosteroids have a role to play in some patients with cancer pain (as they have in non-cancer pain). However, in cancer pain, there are some situations in which destruction of the nervous tissue by the injection of phenol or alcohol may be indicated. In general, this technique may be appropriate if pain is severe and unresponsive to other therapies, if it is relieved by injection of the nerve or nerves with local anaesthetic, and if life expectancy is short. The most commonly used technique is neurolysis of the coeliac plexus in pancreatic cancer, but several other techniques are available. Lesions may also be produced by radiofrequency ablation. The major potential complication is weakness or paralysis caused by damage to adjacent nervous tissue.

Further reading

Allen RR. Neuropathic pain in the cancer patient. *Neurol Clin* 1998;**16**:869–887.

Fine FG. Fentanyl in the treatment of cancer pain. *Semin Oncol* 1997;**24**:20–27.

GilmerHill HS, Boggan JE, Smith KA, Wagner FC. Intrathecal morphine delivered via subcutaneous pump for intractable cancer pain: a review of the literature. *Surg Neurol* 1999;**51**:12–15.

Martin LA, Hagen NA. Neuropathic pain in cancer patients: Mechanisms, syndromes, and clinical controversies. *J Pain Symptom Management* 1997;**14**:99–117.

Mercadante S. Malignant bone pain: pathophysiology and treatment. *Pain* 1997;**69**:1–18.

Payne R. Factors influencing quality of life in cancer patients: the role of transdermal fentanyl in the management of pain. *Semin Oncol* 1998;**25**:47–53.

Ripamonti C, Zecca E, Bruera E. An update on the clinical use of methadone for cancer pain. *Pain* 1997;**70**:109–115.

Twycross R. *Pain relief in advanced cancer.* Churchill Livingstone, 1994.

Pain in children

In the past and to some extent even now, the management of pain in children has been poor. Compared with management of pain in adults, management of pain in children can be more difficult and demanding. Furthermore, children do not always complain in an articulate manner and do not write letters of complaint. However, in recent years, much progress has been made in this area and the myths that surround pain in children have been laid to rest. Such myths include the idea that children are unable to feel pain because of immaturity of the nervous system, the idea that children do not remember pain and the idea that they become addicted to opioids more readily than adults.

Analgesic therapy in children

Pharmacokinetics

Pharmacokinetic values of many drugs in neonates are often different from those in adults and older children. For example, because of differences in drug distribution and immature metabolic pathways, the half-life of opioids is often prolonged by a factor of 2 or 3. However, in children over 1 year of age, the half-life of opioids is often comparable with those of adults. Before prescribing analgesics to children, it is important to be aware of the appropriate age-related dose and any age-specific precautions.

Modes of administration

The oral route is still preferred and some analgesics are available in suspension. Injections should be avoided if possible but intravenous or subcutaneous delivery (via a cannula inserted after application of local anaesthetic cream) may be appropriate, depending on the clinical situation and the choice of drug. Rectal administration is popular if the preparation can be administered during anaesthesia.

Local anaesthetic techniques in children

Local anaesthetic techniques can be used to great advantage in children. Direct application to the skin of preparations such as 4% amethocaine (Ametop) or 2.5% lignocaine with 2.5% prilocaine (Emla) provides excellent surface analgesia. It should be routine practice in all children who require intravenous access or short invasive procedures. Neural blockade (e.g. wound infiltration, nerve blocks, caudal analgesia) is used extensively for postoperative pain relief because the injection can be given during anaesthesia.

Assessment of pain in children

It can be very difficult to assess pain in children but it is important to use a self-reporting method if possible. Clearly, many children cannot understand or use simple categorical or visual analogue pain scoring systems that are appropriate for adults. A face scale is often used; an example is shown in Figure 8. There

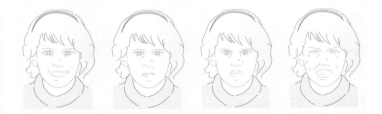

Figure 8 *Example of a face scale for assessment of pain in children.*

are many scales of this type, none of which is perfect. Other more complicated scales are available, but these are used mainly for research purposes (e.g. CHEOPS). Assessment of pain in the neonate is even more difficult but several methods are available (e.g. CRIES, NPS).

Procedural pain in children

Pain and discomfort during invasive therapeutic or investigational procedures should be prevented at all costs in children. If this aspect of care is mismanaged, the child may become severely disturbed and develop a phobia for any future medical attention. If good analgesia cannot be guaranteed during the procedure, the child should be sedated or anaesthetized by an appropriately experienced anaesthetist. Analgesics (paracetamol, NSAIDs, opioids, nerve blocks) should be used appropriately if pain is expected to persist after the procedure.

Psychological approaches to the management of pain in children

Children who experience pain require psychological support, and most of this will come from parents and health-care workers who are involved with day-to-day care. However, in many chronic situations, specialist psychological management is required. This involves a comprehensive psychological appraisal of the situation, including factors such as family problems and the child's overall pain experience. An important theme of psychological intervention is to increase the child's feeling of control and self-confidence. Such intervention may include distraction, participation, relaxation, modelling, desensitization and cognitive behavioural techniques. Appropriately trained and experienced personnel are required for this highly specialized work.

Chronic pain in children

Most chronic pain conditions that occur in adults can occur in children (e.g. phantom limb pain, complex regional pain syndrome, post-traumatic neuropathic pain, juvenile arthritis, cancer pain, postsurgical pain, chronic headache and myofascial pain). Chronic pain in children should be managed aggressively in a multidisciplinary manner. Pain associated with cancer has the additional problem of the need to provide analgesia for interventions such as bone marrow aspiration, venous cannulation and biopsies. Pharmacological management of pain in children is similar to that in adults, including the use of opioids.

Headache is relatively common in childhood and must be investigated thoroughly before symptomatic chronic pain management is started. Migraine is also common. Painful diabetic neuropathy does not usually present until the teenage years. Complex regional pain syndrome is being recognized with increasing frequency in children. Sickle cell disease manifests itself in childhood, and pain management in children with this disease is a considerable challenge. Good pain management is also important in children with haemophilia.

Further reading

AbuSaad HH, Bours GW, Stevens B, Hamers JH. Assessment of pain in the neonate. *Semin Perinatol* 1998;**22**:402–416.

Anderson BJ, Mckee AD, Holford NG. Size, myths and the clinical pharmacokinetics of analgesia in paediatric patients. *Clin Pharmacokinet* 1997;**33**:313–327.

Anonymous. Managing chronic pain in children. *Drug Ther Bull* 1995;**33**:52–55.

Dangel T. Chronic pain management in children. Part I: cancer and phantom pain. *Paediatr Anaesth* 1998;**8**:5–10.

Dangel T. Chronic pain management in children. Part II: reflex sympathetic dystrophy. *Paediatr Anaesth* 1998;**8**:105–112.

Hain RW. Pain scales in children: a review. *Palliative Med* 1997;**11**:341–350.

Royal College of Paediatrics and Child Health. *Prevention and control of pain in children.* London: BMJ Publishing, 1997.

Twycross A, Moriarty A, Betts T. *Paediatric pain management: a multidisciplinary approach.* Oxford: Radcliffe Medical Press, 1998.

Wilkins KL, McGrath PJ, Finley GA, Katz J. Phantom limb sensations and phantom limb pain in child and adolescent amputees. *Pain* 1998;**78**:7–12.

Wolf AR. Pain, nociception and the developing infant. *Paediatr Anaesth* 1999;**9**:7–17.

Index